A Holistic
Approach *to*
ADHD

Deborah Merlin

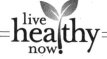

HEALTHY LIVING PUBLICATIONS
Summertown, Tennessee

Cover and interior design: Scattaregia Design

Healthy Living Publications,
a division of Book Publishing Company
P.O. Box 99
Summertown, TN 38483
888-260-8458
bookpubco.com

ISBN: 978-1-57067-319-1

19 18 17 16 15 14   1 2 3 4 5 6 7 8 9

Library of Congress Cataloging-in-Publication Data

Merlin, Deborah.
A holistic approach to ADHD / Deborah Merlin.
    pages cm
ISBN 978-1-57067-319-1 (pbk.) -- ISBN 978-1-57067-886-8 (e-book)
1. Attention-deficit hyperactivity disorder. 2. Attention-deficit hyperactivity disorder--Alternative treatment.
3. Holistic medicine. I. Title.
RJ506.H9M477 2014
618.92'8589--dc23
                    2014026807

Printed on recycled paper

Book Publishing Company is a member of Green Press Initiative. We chose to print this title on paper with 100% post-consumer recycled content, processed without chlorine, which saved the following natural resources:

• 18 trees

• 563 pounds of solid waste

• 8,414 gallons of water

• 1,551 pounds of greenhouse gases

• 8 million BTU of energy

For more information on Green Press Initiative, visit greenpressinitiative.org. Environmental impact estimates were made using the Environmental Defense Fund Paper Calculator. For more information visit papercalculator.org.

CONTENTS

Acknowledgments

Much gratitude is extended to the following experts who have contributed not only to the information in this book but who are also pioneers in the exploration and treatment of ADHD. It is only because of their tireless efforts that we have acquired a wealth of hands-on knowledge, research, testing protocols, and alternative treatment options.

Judith Bluestone

James P. Blumenthal, DC, CCN, DACBN, FABFN

Rashid Buttar, DO, FAAPM, FACAM, FAAIM

Pat Farrell

Stuart H. Garber, DC, PhD

Dan O. Harper, MD, PhD

Janet Starr Hull, PhD

Jack Johnstone, PhD

Kathleen Lewis, DC, CBT

Debbie Lindgren, CIHom

Marlene McKee, Certified Nutrition Educator, DIHom

Trisha Ochoa, CHN

Emily Roberts, MA, LPC-I

Barbara Schwartz, MA

Jane Sheppard

Lesa Werner, ND

Introduction

Among the numerous tough problems affecting our children in this twenty-first century is the unprecedented rise in attention deficit hyperactivity disorder (ADHD). This complex condition is difficult to understand by both parents and the conventional medical community, and that makes it all the more challenging to find effective treatment.

Often parents have an idea that their child may have emotional or behavioral problems because of an erratic behavior. They might have assumed that this was simply their child's kinetic personality coupled with a developing young mind. ADHD is a neurobehavioral disorder associated with difficulty in learning and concentration, inattentive behavior, impulsiveness, and emotional problems.

ADHD is a diagnosis given to 10 percent of all school children in the United States. In 1985, 500,000 children in the United States were diagnosed with ADHD. Today there are between five and seven million. In a class with thirty children, between one and three children are diagnosed with ADHD.

Hyperactivity has existed since the beginning of humankind, but it hasn't always been called the same thing. Various names have been used in the past to describe ADHD and they aren't all bad—think of labels such as enthusiastic, creative, nonconformist, daydreamer, eccentric, high-energy, dedicated, obsessive, type A personality.

So why the name change? No particular reason really. The American Psychiatric Association publishes the official guidelines for naming and diagnosing mental disorders. Their reference book *Diagnostic and Statistical Manual of Mental Disorders* is regularly updated as scientists deal more and more with unidentified modern diseases. Research in the late 1980s began to show changes in "attention deficit," so it was simply renamed for more modern times.

To date, no one has identified the cause for this "mental alteration." Conventional medical treatments consist mainly of various prescription medications. Most of these medications are stimulants, which have the effect of refining focus of thought so that the child can attend to school and homework and not be a disturbance in the classroom. Although these can be effective in some cases, prescription drugs also have many negative side effects that limit their use. However, there are numerous alternative treatments that don't involve drugs or have significant side effects. Among these are nutrition improvement, vitamin supplementation, elimination of foods known to cause allergies, heavy metal detoxification, balancing of neurotransmitters by amino acids, acupuncture, and herbs to help address root causes and then strengthen, build, and repair weakened bodily systems.

The need to educate parents and their children about alternative medicine and lifestyle choices has reached a critical point. I hope you will find some useful answers and helpful resources to explore among these pages.

Food Coloring

I rarely thought twice about food coloring—and when I did, I thought how wonderful it was. Isn't it great that you can make a green cake, decorate Easter eggs, customize treats for children, and make colorful play dough? It seemed as if every label I checked had some type of food coloring in it, so that meant it was safe, right? Unfortunately, the answer turned out to be a resounding no!

Why is it that some children have a bad reaction after eating food that contains coloring? Is it the coloring or something else in the food? Why does one child become hyperactive while another breaks out in a rash? Ben Feingold, a pediatric allergist, made the link between diet, food coloring, and hyperactivity. A number of his patients improved or recovered by changing their diets, specifically by eliminating foods high in salicylates and those that contain colorings.

Artificial food colorings were first introduced after World War II, when the chemical industry joined with the food industry to introduce chemical-based colors, since they were lower in cost than natural colorings and had a longer shelf life. The FDA's website is a valuable database for food coloring information. The site provides precise lists of color ingredients and is quite alarming. You might be horrified to learn, as I was, that all artificial food colorings contain heavy metals, such as lead and mercury, as well as arsenic and myriad chemicals.

One reason this is so disturbing is that one area of the site contains information on the danger of lead contamination and its sources; however, food colorings are not listed as potential sources of exposure. This is especially frightening given all the possibilities for exposure to artificial food colorings in any given day. For example, do your children have sports drinks or fruit juices with coloring? Do their medications contain colorings? What about the macaroni and cheese you made for dinner last night? What are the cumulative effects of this exposure?

Two colorings worth mentioning are not approved for food. The first color, Orange B, is authorized for use only in hot dog and sausage casings. Were you aware that these foods had colorings in them? I certainly was not. Even if you are consciously trying to avoid colorings, you nevertheless have to be extremely vigilant and check every label, because colorings show up in very unexpected places like these.

The second color, Citrus Red No. 2, is approved only for orange skins that are not intended for or used in processing; this means the fresh oranges that we peel and eat. So although we may believe that oranges are a healthy fresh fruit, suitable to offer to our children, they are likely laced with heavy metals.

Artificial colorings are a major concern because not only are they in our food products but they are also present in other daily use items, such as cosmetics, lotions, shampoos, and soaps. Furthermore, the metal allotments for these products are even higher than those allowed in food products.

According to the Children's Environmental Health Project, dermal (skin) absorption is proportional to the concentration of the substance and the surface area to which the substance is applied. Dermal absorption rates vary from person to person and are affected by variables such as skin thickness, occlusions, and the composition of the substance. If a substance is fat soluble, it will be more easily absorbed into the skin.

For these reasons, we must be as vigilant about what we put on our skin as we are about what we eat. In addition, because dermal absorption rates vary from person to person, and the amount of toxic substances vary from product to product, people will be affected differently by various products. Doing something as innocent as washing your hands with soap could expose you to more than you bargained for.

In addition to identifying a link between food colorings and hyperactivity, Dr. Feingold noticed a marked increase in ADHD classifications after the mass introduction of food colorings into our society. If lead has been implicated in ADHD (see page 11), and colorings have lead in them, then removing added colorings from our diets and environment is crucial.

The *Journal of Developmental & Behavioral Pediatrics* published information regarding fifteen trials with 219 children; all were double-blind, crossover trials. When just artificial food colorings were eliminated from the children's diets, the children's behavior improved significantly. Furthermore, the dietary removal of food colorings produced one-third to one-half the improvement typically seen with ADHD medication therapy.

It is instructive to consider how saturated with artificial colorings most ADHD medications are. For example, Ritalin contains D&C Yellow No. 10; Strattera contains FD&C Blue No. 2, synthetic iron oxide, and edible black ink; and Dexedrine contains FD&C Yellow No. 5 and No. 6.

Children taking these drugs are being exposed to lead, arsenic, and mercury, among many other toxins. Parents also need to be extremely careful with whatever medications they give their children, including acetaminophen, ibuprofen, and antibiotics, and ensure that alternative products don't contain food dyes. As parents, we can check food labels, but we must rely on physicians to select our medicines, since the bottles provided by pharmacists don't list all of the ingredients. Homeopathic products and supplements may provide safer alternatives (see page 40).

Most parents are completely unaware of the colorings used in their food, cosmetic products, and medicines. Some who are aware are shocked to find out that colorings do not come from natural substances. Here are a few surprising examples of food and personal care products that contain food colorings:

- Bathtime Colorblast Tablets: FD&C Blue No. 1, D&C Red No. 33, FD&C Yellow No. 5
- Flintstones Vitamins: aspartame, FD&C Red No. 40 Aluminum Lake, FD&C Yellow No. 6 Aluminum Lake, FD&C Blue No. 2
- Gatorade Fruit Punch: FD&C Red No. 40
- Johnson's Baby Shampoo: D&C Yellow No. 10, D&C Orange No. 4
- M&Ms (plain): FD&C Blue No. 1, FD&C Blue No. 1 Aluminum Lake, FD&C Blue No. 2 Aluminum Lake, FD&C Red No. 40, FD&C Red No. 40 Aluminum Lake, FD&C Yellow No. 5, FD&C Yellow No. 6
- Pampers Hand Soap: FD&C Yellow No. 5, D&C Green No. 5, FD&C Orange No. 4

We do not know the cumulative effects of regular exposure to food and cosmetic colorings. We also do not know how food colorings interact with each other and with other toxic substances. I have found no studies regarding this, and that alone is alarming.

Cleaning products present an interesting challenge, since manufacturers do not have to identify the ingredients of their products on the labels. Material Safety Data Sheets (MSDS) are available for consumers to view via most companies' websites. Although manufacturers are required to provide information on the MSDS regarding established exposure limits, they are not required to provide an ingredient or coloring list because their formulations are protected by patent laws.

So what can we do? The first step is to remove colorings from our environment. Although this might appear difficult because colorings are so pervasive, there are easy options and alternatives. For example, if you want to color a cake frosting or homemade play dough, look in your natural food store for packaged colorings made from real foods, such as turmeric, blue-berries, and beets. You can also make your own natural colorings by adding these foods to whatever it is you want to dye. Natural food stores also carry a variety of foods, personal care products, nonprescription medications, and cleaners that do not contain colorings.

Preparing as many meals as possible from scratch at home is also a step in the right direction, because that way you can control what you put in your food. If you need to obtain medication and are not sure if it contains colorings, you can check online at the Internet Drug Index (rxlist.com). If your medication is made with colorings, contact a compounding pharmacy to see if the pharmacist can compound it without the added colors. A list of compounding pharmacies can be found at the the International Academy of Compounding Pharmacists website (iacprx.org).

Lead, Mercury, and Arsenic

A study performed by the National Academy of Sciences (NAS) contends that roughly 3 percent of all developmental and neurological disorders in the United States are caused by toxic chemicals and other environmental contaminants. The same study showed that environmental triggers, along with a genetic predisposition, may cause approximately 25 percent of developmental and neurological deficits. The NAS also acknowledged that the study was only referring to well-recognized and clinically diagnosed mental and physical disabilities, and therefore the 25 percent estimate may in fact be higher.

Children's vulnerability derives from both rapid development and incomplete defense systems:

- A developing child's chemical exposures are greater pound for pound than those of adults.
- An immature, porous blood-brain barrier allows greater chemical exposures to the developing brain.

- Children have lower levels of some chemical-binding proteins, allowing more of a chemical to reach target organs.
- A baby's organs and systems are rapidly developing, and therefore they are often more vulnerable to damage from chemical exposure.
- Bodily systems that detoxify and excrete industrial chemicals are not yet fully developed.
- The longer future life span of a child compared to an adult allows more time for adverse effects to arise.

Lead

Many people are not aware that the symptoms of lead poisoning and heavy metal toxicity can mimic the symptoms of other childhood conditions, such as ADHD. In addition, several studies also point to a link between lead poisoning and ADHD. One that was published in the journal *Environmental Health Perspectives* showed that children with blood lead levels of more than 2 micrograms of lead per deciliter were four times more likely to be diagnosed with ADHD than children with levels below 0.8 micrograms per deciliter. The acceptable blood level for lead, according to the government, is 10 micrograms per deciliter. The study estimates that more than five million children between the ages of four and fifteen in the United States have levels higher than 2 micrograms per deciliter.

The American Academy of Child and Adolescent Psychiatry estimates that one out of every six children in the United States has blood lead levels in the toxic range. Lead exposure has been linked to developmental delays, peripheral neuropathy, altered thyroid hormone, and reduced fertility. In elderly adults, levels over 4 mcg can have neurobehavioral effects.

Several studies have been done on the dermal absorption of lead. One study concluded that significant amounts of inorganic lead compounds can be absorbed through the skin; therefore, protection should always be used. Another study evaluated the effectiveness of skin cleansers at removing lead from the skin. The results show it's necessary to prevent skin contamination from occurring in the first place, because just brief contact allows for penetration, even when it is quickly followed by washing.

Mercury

When we get a cavity, some dentists will fill our teeth with amalgams that contain mercury. Mercury has been implicated in autism, ADHD, learning disabilities, endocrine problems, allergies, asthma, rheumatoid arthritis, and a host of other disorders. According to the FDA, toxicity of mercury compounds is extensively documented in scientific literature. Mercury compounds are readily absorbed through unbroken skin, through the lungs by inhalation, and by intestinal absorption after ingestion. Mercury is absorbed from topical applications and is accumulated in the body, giving rise to numerous adverse effects. Additionally, microorganisms in the environment can convert various forms of mercury into highly toxic methylmercury, which has been found in the food supply and is considered a serious environmental problem.

Common Dreams Newswire reported in 2004 that Environmental Protection Agency scientists using data collected by the Centers for Disease Control estimated that one in six pregnant women has enough mercury in her blood to pose a risk of brain damage to her developing child. Lower levels of mercury can lead to a variety of symptoms, including fever, insomnia, rapidly changing moods, and tremors.

The reason some individuals suffer severe damage from mercury when others don't is due to variable factors such as biological individuality and genetic predisposition. In addition, the type of exposure—inhalation, digestion, injection, or dermal (skin)—makes an enormous difference. It also matters what type of mercury exposure the individual received—organic or inorganic mercury—and if organic, whether it was ethylmercury or methylmercury. Other factors include the following:

- The frequency of exposure to the source of toxicity.
- Whether there was exposure from the mother before birth.

- Whether the mother was inoculated or had RhoGAM either during pregnancy or prior to conception.
- The number of vaccine administrations and over what period of time.
- Exposure through diet.
- The proximity to industrial sites and exposure to fossil fuel pollution.

The only solution for children who cannot eliminate mercury from their bodies on their own is to administer effective treatments for removing the mercury while repairing and enhancing their immune systems.

Arsenic

Arsenic poisoning has been linked to developmental, cardiovascular, neurological, and respiratory issues. It has also been associated with cancer. In fact, an increased risk of skin cancer in humans has been connected with chronic exposure to inorganic arsenic via medications, contaminated water, and the workplace.

Arsenic is present in foods such as meat, fish, and poultry, and according to the Department of Health and Human Services, our dietary intake accounts for 80 percent of our exposure. (Note that fish arsenic has a low toxicity in humans and is excreted rapidly in our urine). Fungicides, herbicides, insecticides, paints, and water are other sources of arsenic exposure.

According to the Department of Health and Human Services, dermal absorption of arsenic is low, but arsenic is readily absorbed if inhaled or ingested. Many wood-based playground structures have been removed out of the fear that children would touch the arsenic-treated wood and then put their hands in their mouths.

A study of 201 children under the age of ten concluded that as little as .0017 milligrams of arsenic per day affected children's performance in tasks that required switching attention. When the exposure increased to .0034 milligrams per day, the children showed decreased performance in tasks that involved switching attention as well as in tests that measured memory.

Artificial Sweeteners

Can ADHD be caused by artificial sweeteners? You bet. Just look around. The increases in ADHD (and the label itself) are perfectly timed with the introduction of the artificial sweetener aspartame in such products as NutraSweet and Equal in 1981.

Diana Dow-Edwards of SUNY Health Science Center in Brooklyn investigated evidence of intellectual and developmental disabilities in laboratory guinea pigs by administering aspartame to them during pregnancy. Since brain development occurs in the womb in both guinea pigs and humans, the results of her investigations could be extrapolated to people.

Dow-Edwards' research evaluated the harmful influences of moderate doses of aspartame administered to pregnant mothers, especially those with liver problems, because all chemical sweeteners are metabolized in the liver. She concluded from her studies that using moderate quantities of aspartame during pregnancy could produce a dramatic increase in the number of offspring born with diminished brain function. Not only does this study call into question the use of aspartame, but it also challenges the use of sweetener blends, such as those that combine aspartame and sucralose. Where aspartame penetrates, so follows the chlorine in sucralose. Corporate marketers claim that the chlorine atoms in sucralose (which goes by the brand name Splenda) are so tightly bound they do not break down inside the body, but when sucralose is blended with aspartame, the chlorine in sucralose can be ushered into the brain alongside its chemical counterpart.

As early as 1970, John Olney, a research psychiatrist in the Department of Psychiatry at Washington University School of Medicine, pioneered proof of aspartame's dangerous entry into the brain. He informed G.D. Searle and Company (the developer of aspartame and founder of The NutraSweet Company), warning them that the aspartic acid in aspartame caused holes to form in the brains of laboratory mice. Olney proved that excess aspartic acid in the brain destroys brain neurons. He established that approximately 75 percent of the neural cells in any particular area of the brain could be killed before any clinical symptoms of a chronic illness are even noticed.

Russell L. Blaylock, a professor of neurosurgery at the University of Mississippi Medical Center, provides over five hundred scientific references in his book *Excitotoxins: The Taste that Kills*, proving that excess free excitatory amino acids (such as the aspartic acid and phenylalanine found in aspartame) cause serious chronic neurological disorders along with a host of acute physical symptoms. The FDA has recorded in their files the following mental symptoms related to aspartame use: anxiety attacks, depression, fatigue, headaches and migraines, sleep problems, and vision problems.

The evidence is clear that artificial sweeteners negatively affect the human brain. In this ever-continuing web of confusion over which chemicals are causing which health reactions, it is wise to return to natural sweeteners and whole foods, especially during pregnancy and during childhood development.

Vaccinations

The vaccine decision is one of the most important choices we make as parents. Increasingly, childhood vaccines are implicated as the cause of growing rates of autism and ADHD. However, in questioning vaccines, we open ourselves up to a great deal of criticism, disapproval, and accusations of child neglect from doctors, school administrators, public health officials, family members, and other parents. How, they ask, do we dare question a practice that has prevented so many devastating diseases and saved so many lives? Aren't we putting our child and other children at risk for contracting serious diseases? After all, the government agencies designated to protect public health and most doctors say that childhood vaccines are safe.

If you dig a little deeper into the issue, you'll find many gaps and limitations in the data and knowledge regarding vaccine safety. Vaccines are capable of causing serious damage. Because they contain lab-altered viruses, bacteria, and toxic substances, vaccines have the ability to cause mild to severe neurological and immunological damage or even death, depending on the vaccine given, the combination of vaccines given, the health of the child at the time of vaccination, and the genetic or biological factors that predispose the child to this damage. Vaccines are potent, toxic drugs that contain aluminum, antibiotics, formaldehyde, mercury, and other dangerous, harmful components. Thoughtful parents are beginning to question the practice of injecting these toxic substances into the bodies of small babies and artificially manipulating their fragile immune systems during the crucial time of brain and immune development.

No Long-Term or Real-World Safety Studies

Pharmaceutical companies do safety testing of vaccines, but long-term studies are not done. The follow-up for vaccine safety testing on individuals before a vaccine is marketed is only a few weeks or a couple of months at most. Pharmaceutical companies and government health officials rely on post-marketing data to see if there are reports of serious side effects and reactions after the vaccine has been released and given to millions of children. But most doctors are reluctant to report adverse reactions, and it is estimated that between only 1 and 10 percent of vaccine reactions are ever reported. Even so, between twelve thousand and fourteen thousand adverse reactions, including hospitalizations, injuries, and death, are reported annually to the Vaccine Adverse Event Reporting System. Since it may be difficult to establish causal relationship, many of the reported reactions are dismissed as coincidental with no further study.

The control groups for determining adverse reactions are not unvaccinated children. Instead, they are children who have received other vaccines. This makes it possible for the vaccine in question to appear safer than it actually may be. In addition, no adequate studies have ever been done on the real-world risk—the cumulative effect of multiple doses of numerous vaccines given in the first five years of life.

Chronic Diseases Rise as Vaccinations Increase

Chronic diseases and disabilities in children have risen dramatically as vaccination rates for a growing number of vaccines climb higher than ever before. Twenty-five years ago, children following the recommended vaccine schedule received twenty-three doses of seven vaccines before age six. Today's children get forty-eight doses of fourteen vaccines by age six. With the additional recommendation for annual flu shots, children may now get sixty-nine doses of sixteen vaccines by age eighteen.

Given all these vaccinations, are our children healthier? Health officials continue to insist that there is no connection between vaccines and autism. However, Bernadine Healy, former head of the National Institutes of Health and a member of the Institute of Medicine, stated that public health officials have intentionally avoided researching the link between vaccines and autism because they are afraid the answer will scare the public. She acknowledged that public health officials have failed to fully research vaccines and how they may contribute to autism. Dr. Healy, along with many other medical doctors, believed there may be a subset of children who, for genetic or other reasons, are susceptible to developing autism following vaccination.

In June 2007, the first-ever investigation to determine the difference between vaccinated and unvaccinated children was done by Generation Rescue, a parent-funded nonprofit organization. This survey of over seventeen thousand children compared the rates of ADHD, autism, and asthma between vaccinated and unvaccinated children. Results showed that vaccinated US children have a significantly higher risk of neurological disorders—including autism and ADHD—than unvaccinated children. This was not a comprehensive enough study to confirm a connection, but it certainly raises a rather large red flag and demonstrates the need for a national study to compare outcomes between vaccinated and unvaccinated children.

Toxicity of Vaccines

A growing number of doctors believe that a baby's immune system is not strong enough to handle the amount of vaccines typically given, and their livers and kidneys are not developed enough to metabolize or excrete the toxic chemicals and heavy metals in vaccines. Parents should know that even though mercury has finally been taken out of most childhood vaccines, there is still a significant amount of mercury in many flu shots as well as tetanus booster shots and some meningitis vaccines. Trace amounts of mercury still remain in other vaccines. Mercury is known to be one of the most toxic substances on the planet, and no amount of mercury is safe, especially when injected into a baby's small, developing body.

Even though most of the recent discussion concerning toxicity of vaccines has revolved around the mercury issue, mercury is certainly not the only toxicity problem with childhood vaccines. Aluminum is used as an adjuvant to boost the immune response of vaccines. Scientific evidence of the safety of injected aluminum is sorely lacking. Aluminum is a heavy metal that can accumulate in tissues and build up to toxic levels in the bloodstream, bones, and brain. Accumulation of aluminum in the brain is known to impair neurological and mental development. Animal studies show that aluminum causes convulsions and impairs memory and learning.

The difference in the amount of aluminum that may be considered safe for babies and the amount that is actually contained in vaccines is alarming. The FDA website says that premature babies receiving injected aluminum through intravenous fluids at levels greater than 4 to 5 micrograms per kilogram of body weight per day can accumulate aluminum at levels associated with central nervous system and bone toxicity, and toxic buildup may occur at even lower rates. For a tiny premature baby, the toxic dose would be 10 to 20 micrograms. It is estimated that a twelve-pound, two-month-old, full-term healthy baby could safely receive at least 30 micrograms of intra-venously injected aluminum per day. But it is unknown how much more aluminum a healthy baby could handle and how much could be safely injected into a baby via vaccines. The safety of aluminum in vaccines has never been established. No research has been done to determine a baby's ability to excrete aluminum to prevent toxic buildup. No one has measured the levels of aluminum absorption by the bloodstream when an aluminum-containing vaccine is injected into a baby. Also disturbing is the lack of data to determine if injected aluminum interacts with other vaccine toxins to cause harm to small, developing bodies.

A newborn baby receiving a hepatitis B shot on his first day of life gets 250 micrograms of aluminum from this vaccine. The total amount of aluminum that a two-month-old baby receives from the recommended "well-baby" vaccines could vary from 295 to 1,225 micrograms, depending on which vaccines are given. This dose is usually repeated at four months and again at six months of age.

Vaccines also contain various animal products and are created using both human and animal tissues. These tissues can contain viruses and other contaminants. Even though there are processes to detoxify and clean the vaccines, some viruses have still made it into the final vaccine products that were injected into babies. One well-known case was a monkey virus known to cause cancer that was found in the polio vaccine given to millions of babies during the 1950s and 1960s. There remains a possibility of an unknown or new virus that may not be detected with current testing.

Vaccine Reactions

Vaccine reactions can take many forms, including one or more of the following:

- brain inflammation
- bruising
- collapse and shock

- death
- difficulty breathing or wheezing
- dizziness
- excessive sleepiness or lack of responsiveness
- high fever
- hives
- itching
- mental and/or physical regression
- muscle weakness or limpness
- paleness or changes in skin or lip color
- prolonged crying (especially high-pitched screaming in infants)
- rapid heartbeat
- rash
- seizures or convulsions (shaking, twitching, jerking)
- swelling, redness, and pain at the injection site
- unusual irritability or other behavior changes
- vomiting or diarrhea

Many parents have reported that their baby had a high-pitched scream for many hours directly after receiving a vaccine and then regressed developmentally, eventually being diagnosed with autism months later. Some babies have died after being vaccinated.

Weakened Immunity

A growing number of doctors agree that weakened immunity and susceptibility to allergies, asthma, and chronic infections is another long-term consequence of the large number of vaccines given to babies and children at their most vulnerable time of immune development. A baby's immune system develops through breastfeeding and proper nutrition and from its complex responses to natural exposure to disease. When a baby is naturally exposed to a virus, the immune system has several layers of responses that deal with the invasion. Allowing the range of acute inflammatory responses to typical childhood diseases strengthens immunity and strengthens the child's health overall.

Conversely, injecting multiple doses of altered viruses and toxins directly into the body bypasses many of the normal immune responses. The vaccine injection triggers antibody production, but antibodies are only one level of protection and not full natural immunity. The immune system is very complex, and the different branches of the immune system require a balanced, synergistic relationship to function properly. Repeated vaccinations may overstimulate the branch that produces antibodies while suppressing the branch responsible for acute inflammatory responses.

Intelligent doctors and parents are beginning to question this manipulation of the immune system. Because we are seeing a huge increase in pediatric allergies, asthma, autoimmune diseases, and chronic immune deficiencies, we must look at a mass vaccination policy and demand the proper studies to find out what is happening to our children's immune systems.

Universal Vaccines for Everyone?

Does it make sense to mandate vaccines for every child given the risks involved? The public health strategy for eliminating diseases includes universal vaccines for everyone, regardless of risks to the individual child, who may have biological or genetic susceptibility to vaccine damage. There are no tests that can show which babies will have serious reactions. Some children must be sacrificed in order to achieve the goal of eradicating disease in a population. The government, health organizations, schools, and physicians tell us that more lives will be lost to a disease if we don't vaccinate against it. But is this statement really true in the current reality of high-tech medicine in a population with effective sanitation and knowledge about the immunology of breastfeeding?

We cannot wipe out every disease on the planet. It may be more sensible to focus on naturally strengthening our children's immune systems to effectively deal with the increasing number of superbugs created by the inappropriate and massive use of antibiotics than to inject numerous toxins into their delicate, developing bodies. If we allow our children's immune systems to develop as nature intended through breastfeeding, good nutrition, and other natural immune-enhancing methods, then it doesn't make sense to inject them with foreign materials and toxins that can weaken their health, especially since the safety of these injections may be questionable. An increasing number of parents are not willing to take the risk of sacrificing their children to a point of view that goes against their core beliefs about health and wellness.

The Captive, Multibillion-Dollar Vaccine Market

What fuels the ubiquitous belief that vaccines are the supreme solution to disease and that those who do not accept vaccines are putting themselves and others at risk? The vaccine industry is money driven and uses the government, doctors, and school officials to effectively market their products and gain mass acceptance of their message. The Food and Drug Administration (FDA) accepts safety data from the manufacturers and licenses vaccines used in the United States. After a vaccine is licensed, the Advisory Committee on Immunization Practices (ACIP), appointed by the Centers for Disease Control (CDC), makes recommendations on dosages and age ranges for children. ACIP immunization recommendations are extremely influential and enacted into law as mandates by individual states. In the past twenty-five years, every childhood vaccine produced by the drug companies has been mandated for use by all US children.

Many members of both the ACIP and the FDA's advisory committees have been found by the Committee on Oversight and Government Reform to have blatant conflicts of interest, with strong financial ties to the pharmaceutical companies that make vaccines. The Committee exposed these conflicts of interest, focusing on the approval of the rotavirus vaccine, which was found to cause severe bowel obstructions.

This vaccine was pulled from the market after a significant number of babies were injured and required surgery and one baby died from the vaccine. It was found that the FDA's advisory committee members, who approved the rotavirus vaccine, were aware of the problems but voted to approve it anyway. Three out of these five members had financial ties to the pharmaceutical companies that were developing different versions of the rotavirus vaccine. This is not an isolated incident. Congressman Dan Burton, the head of the Reform Committee at the time, remarked, "If the panels that have made the decisions on all vaccines on the Childhood Immunization Schedule had as many conflicts as we found with rotavirus, then the entire process has been polluted and the public trust has been violated."

A mandate for every child in the country to use their vaccines gives the manufacturers a steady and constant demand for their products. And since they are protected from legal action by the Vaccine Injury Compensation Program of 1986, they are rushing to bring new vaccines to market. Vaccines are the only commercial products marketed and sold for profit in the United States that are not subject to product liability laws.

As more parents are beginning to mistrust vaccines, money is being spent to fund pro-vaccine organizations for public relations and damage control. Vaccine "experts" are hired to manipulate public opinion by denying the severity of adverse reactions and reinforcing the belief that the benefits of vaccines outweigh the risks. Instead of becoming alarmed by reports of vaccine-induced brain damage and pushing for the unbiased research needed to determine why this is happening, vaccine manufacturers and government agencies embark on intensive public-relations campaigns to make sure the public trust in vaccines has not been diminished in any way. Their main goal is to keep the vaccine program moving forward at any cost.

Parents Can Make Informed Choices

At the doctor's office, parents are given a two-page "Vaccine Information Statement," which highlights the importance of vaccines and downplays the harmful effects. Many parents are coerced into vaccinating their children by doctors who say they will no longer accept their children as patients if they are not vaccinated. Many parents are also worried that their children will be denied school attendance if they don't vaccinate.

Informed consent means that an informed patient (or parent) has absolute freedom to accept or reject any specific medical treatment or procedure. The patient (or parent) has the right to be treated sensitively and compassionately while learning about his or her options. The doctor is both ethically obligated and legally required to participate in a communication process that helps the patient to understand the risks and benefits as well as become aware of alternatives. There are informed consent statutes and case laws in all fifty states in the United States. Why don't these revered informed consent laws apply when it comes to vaccinations, especially when this medical intervention carries the risk of brain damage and death? Parents are almost never told about exemptions to state vaccine laws. They are usually told they do not have a choice.

We have the right to select the kind of preventive health care that is appropriate for our families. We should never be forced to accept any medical procedure that carries the risk of injury or death against our will. Making an informed decision requires that we evaluate the needs of our families and assess the pros and cons of each vaccine within this context. If we wish to take the precautionary approach and keep our children's bodies free from harmful toxins so they can develop healthy immunity naturally, we have every right to say no to vaccines.

In the United States, we have the legal right to exempt our children from vaccines and still have them attend public school. All states have medical exemptions (these must be signed by a doctor), forty-eight states have exemptions for religious beliefs, and fifteen states have exemptions for philosophical beliefs. Claiming the philosophical exemption in some states (California, for example) is as easy as signing the statement on the back of the school's vaccination record or providing a letter that states that vaccinations are against your personal beliefs. When you claim an exemption, there should be no questions and your child legally must be admitted to school. A religious exemption can be a little trickier, sometimes requiring a letter from a recognized church, but in many cases parents can write a letter simply stating that vaccinations are against their religious beliefs.

If you are seeking an exemption, get a copy of your state's immunization law and follow exactly what it says about what is needed for an exemption. Many parents are not aware that these exemptions exist, since public health officials, doctors, and school administrators usually don't mention them.

We need to realize that our parental rights have been stripped in the process of trying to eradicate disease, and this has been done in ways that can have devastating consequences to our children's health and well-being. We blindly put our faith in the medical industry and public health officials, who view disease as an enemy to exterminate at all costs, regardless of the number of damaged children or deaths that may occur in the process. When we accept these policies, we give our power over to the government and the vaccine industry, and we let them intrude in our family's private health care choices.

We, as parents, need to take our power back and make informed choices for our children without coercion, threat, or disapproval by doctors or health officials. And we should be applauded, not shamed, by our friends, family, and other parents for refusing to blindly follow "doctor's orders" as we carefully consider all the issues that can affect the health of our precious children. In fact, thorough investigation before making vaccine decisions and parental demand for proven safety are the only things that will ever begin to make disease prevention safe for everyone's children.

Gluten and Dairy

Allergies to wheat, gluten, and dairy products are surprisingly common among children and adults suffering from the symptoms of ADHD. Removing the foods that cause the allergic reaction can have enormous beneficial results.

"Bread is the staff of life" is a common refrain, and bread and grains are so highly valued worldwide that the word "bread" is sometimes used to refer to food in general, as in the phrase "breaking bread." Most every culture believes that bread and grains should occupy the center of a nutritious diet. Unfortunately, this belief could not be further from the truth; in fact, grain foods are likely partially at fault for many chronic diseases that affect society. While it is true that a diet high in grains will prevent someone from starving to death, it will not allow him or her to maintain or achieve good health.

Anthropological evidence shows that grains have only been a part of the human diet for about twelve thousand years, originating in the Middle East, where populations were among the first to farm grains. Among Aboriginal and American Indian populations, grains have been consumed for only a few hundred years. In the grand scheme of things, this is a very short period of time, particularly when we consider that this is the amount of time the complex human body has had to adapt to this new food. Grains were unlike any source of nutrition that humans had been eating up until that point; the diet of early humans consisted mainly of vegetables, fruits, nuts, and meats, which we had evolved to eat over the course of many millions of years. Therefore, it is not surprising that so many of us have difficulty properly digesting them.

Recent discoveries using DNA analysis have shown that as humans began farming grains, their stature changed dramatically. In fact, over the course of only a few generations, our agricultural ancestors decreased in height by five to six inches while their head circumference, a marker correlated with brain size, decreased by 11 percent. Amazingly, this happened after only a few generations of eating a diet high in grains.

Further exacerbating the negative effects that grains have on our bodies is the fact that our agricultural practices are constantly forcing grains to evolve further. This usually entails creating grains with higher protein content to allow them to reproduce more quickly and in harsher climates. When we change the nutrient profiles of these foods, our bodies are further taxed in their efforts to fully adapt to them and learn how to use them properly.

Malabsorption and Inflammation

Digestion is a somewhat complex process that begins with the chewing of food and continues when the food is chemically broken down by specific digestive enzymes. The process ends when the food is fully broken down and absorbed through the gastrointestinal wall into the bloodstream. Only when these processes are completed can we use the nutrients in our foods to fuel our bodies and minds.

Gluten, the protein in wheat and related grains (including barley, rye, oats, spelt, Kamut, and triticale) is particularly difficult to fully digest. Gluten is held together by sulfide bonds, which are very difficult to break. For this reason, gluten is only ever partially digested. Moreover, gluten-containing grains have enzyme inhibitors, which interfere with protein breakdown, further reducing the body's ability to digest these grains properly. Eating gluten-containing foods frequently may exhaust the body's enzyme supplies, exacerbating poor digestion.

Dairy products, particularly homogenized dairy products, are also difficult for many people to digest because of the substances created during this process. Since proteins in gluten-containing grains and dairy products are not fully broken down, they wreak havoc on the digestive system. Not only are the nutrients from these foods not absorbed, but gluten-containing grains and dairy products also have other more detrimental and long-lasting effects.

The most devastating effects of gluten and dairy malabsorption are found within the immune system. Approximately 60 percent of our immune system resides in our gastrointestinal tract. This portion of our immune system is called gut-associated lymphoid tissue (GALT), and it serves as our first defense against an attack on our body. This tissue launches the first assault against the common cold, kills bacteria that finds its way into our food, and combats toxins from our environment. We are bombarded by bacteria, viruses, chemicals, and other antigens, but a healthy gastrointestinal tract fights these predators without us even knowing it. We only feel the effects of these toxins if they make it past this first defense. For this reason, the health of our gastrointestinal tract is paramount to overall good health.

When we consume a diet containing gluten and dairy, we are directly contributing to poor gastrointestinal health due to the poor digestion of these foods. When gluten and dairy proteins aren't broken down as a result of inadequate enzymes, enzyme inhibitors, or other factors, these proteins remain in the gastrointestinal tract as large particles. This wouldn't be so bad if these particles were excreted. Instead, GALT gets involved and attempts to determine what these larger proteins are. Since it cannot properly categorize these particles, it treats them as predators, or toxins, and launches an immune attack against them.

The immune attack process results in irritation of the gastrointestinal tract. The tissues get inflamed in the same way that the mucous membranes of your nose get inflamed when you have a cold or flu. In addition, they release a protective mucous layer to prevent absorption of the toxin, similar to how your nose runs when you have a cold. This process wouldn't be problematic if it only occurred a few times a year, like a cold or flu; when it occurs very regularly, however, it becomes troublesome.

The average American eats at least one, and often many more, gluten- or dairy-containing foods every day; it is estimated that 19 percent of the American diet is composed of gluten-containing foods. That means this process is affecting most Americans to one degree or another almost every day.

Leaky Gut Syndrome

When your gastrointestinal tract is in a constant state of inflammation, you develop a condition called leaky gut syndrome. This condition is very common in children with ADHD, autism, allergies, chemical sensitivities, and many chronic illnesses.

Leaky gut is characterized as a combination of both underabsorption and overabsorption within the gastrointestinal tract. When the gut becomes inflamed as a result of an immune attack, it becomes more permeable and less able to properly mediate the passage of particles into the bloodstream. As a result, food particles that have not been fully broken down are allowed to pass out of the intestine and into the bloodstream at points of inflammation. In addition, increased mucus within the gut blocks the absorption of digested food particles where the mucus is present.

While it may seem counterintuitive that a leaky gut allows large particles into the bloodstream and blocks small particles, the effects can be illustrated by one of the common diagnostic tests for this condition. Leaky gut syndrome is often diagnosed by administering a lactulose-mannitol test. During this test, you drink a solution containing mannitol and lactulose and then collect your urine over a period of time. Mannitol is made up of small molecules that should be very easily absorbed from the intestinal tract and excreted in urine, while lactulose is made up of larger molecules that are not normally absorbed and, as a result, are excreted in feces. For a person with a healthy gastrointestinal tract, the amount of mannitol in the urine should be high and lactulose should be very low or nonexistent. With leaky gut syndrome, the amount of lactulose in the urine is much higher, while mannitol levels can vary depending on the severity of the case. Consequently, large, poorly absorbed molecules are absorbed and, depending on the severity of mucus production, small, easily absorbed molecules are not absorbed. This pattern extends to all substances that enter the gastrointestinal tract.

When undigested food particles and other foreign substances are allowed to enter the bloodstream, they can trigger other immune responses that affect the entire body, not just the gut. This leads to hypersensitivity to foods, the environment, and normally benign substances.

Cerebral allergies are a typical consequence of this immune response, and wheat and milk are the most common culprits. Cerebral allergies are the basis of allergy-addiction cycles, where the body craves certain allergens to avoid withdrawal symptoms. With leaky gut syndrome, certain antigens or antigen-antibody complexes enter the bloodstream and then cross the blood-brain barrier and negatively affect brain health. Common symptoms include anxiety, irritability, aggression, and even psychotic episodes. This phenomenon is very common in children because they often eat very limited diets with little variety.

The gastrointestinal tract not only works to break down food and allow its absorption, it also serves as the body's first barrier against attacks from foreign molecules. It protects against bacteria, chemicals, fungi, heavy metals, viruses, and any other particles that might find their way into your body via the GI tract. With increased gastrointestinal permeability, these particles are more readily absorbed. This can lead to chronic bacterial, fungal, and viral infections; heavy metal poisoning; and chemical sensitivities, among other health problems. Some of these toxins are even able to cross the blood-brain barrier and wreak havoc within the central nervous system. This is particularly noteworthy in the case of heavy metal poisoning because of the extensive harm that heavy metals can have on the nervous system.

Any toxin that enters the body, and many endogenous chemicals (such as hormones and inflammation complexes) made within the body, need to be detoxified before they can be safely excreted. This detoxification occurs primarily within the liver and mucous membranes, and relies upon certain enzymes, nutrients, and biochemical processes, collectively referred to as detoxification pathways. The body's ability to eliminate these toxins and endogenous chemicals is limited by its supply of the necessary enzymes and nutrients. Therefore, when the toxin level exceeds the capacity of the detoxification pathways, toxins enter into the bloodstream, accumulate, and damage the body. This phenomenon is often referred to as the "rain barrel effect," where the body is doing just fine as toxins accumulate, but once they completely fill the "rain barrel" and begin to flow over, health problems ensue. Once your "rain barrel" is full, your detoxification pathways are at their limit, and toxins are now able to wreak havoc on your body.

With leaky gut syndrome, not only do greater levels of toxins enter the bloodstream, but along with them high levels of inflammatory immune complexes are delivered to the liver. This stresses the body's detoxification pathways further, allowing an even greater number of toxins into the bloodstream. The likelihood of these toxins entering the brain and nervous system increases greatly at this point, and the body's ability to detoxify is simultaneously diminished because of the increased toxic load on the liver. This vicious cycle of accumulating toxins creates an overall decrease in health.

Chronic infections, elevated heavy metal levels, and chemical sensitivities often coexist in cases of ADHD. The symptoms of ADHD often reverse when these other conditions are removed. Therefore, addressing these toxins is paramount to healing, and the first step is addressing the increased permeability of the gastrointestinal tract and stopping these antigens from being reintroduced into the body.

Thankfully, leaky gut syndrome is reversible. The process of reversal involves allowing the gut to heal so that it can return to normal functioning. This usually requires several steps and can take months, but the results are quite amazing.

The first step always involves removing the offending foods from the diet. For most of my clients that means avoiding all gluten-containing foods and usually avoiding dairy products as well. This stops the immune attack that begins in the gut and allows the GI tract to heal. The process of healing can be monitored with follow-up lactulose-mannitol tests showing a return to healthy levels. When patients watch their progress, it often provides them with the necessary motivation to continue with this step, which is by far the most difficult. When working with children, it is especially important to find replacements for the foods that are being removed from their diets. Fortunately, so many people are avoiding these foods these days that alternatives can be found at most natural food stores. Rice-based breads and pastas serve as excellent substitutes for their gluten-containing counterparts, and nut-based milks and cheeses, also available at most natural food stores, are good replacements for similar dairy products. Soy milk and soy-based cheeses are another option, although children may prefer the taste and texture of the nut-based alternatives.

A Four-Pronged Approach

Beyond removing the offending foods, taking full-spectrum digestive enzymes with each meal can be quite beneficial, as they help with the breakdown of all foods. Each enzyme targets a particular food type and assists in its breakdown. For example, amylase digests amylose, a type of carbohydrate, but it does not digest lactose, a different type of carbohydrate, nor does it digest lipids or proteins. Full-spectrum digestive enzymes contain protein-digesting enzymes, such as papain and various proteases, along with the fat-digesting enzyme lipase, and a number of carbohydrate-digesting enzymes, such as amylase and invertase. These enzymes provide additional digestive assistance and increase the likelihood that your food will be in the appropriately digested state by the time it is absorbed. In addition to augmenting your naturally occurring enzymes, full-spectrum digestive enzymes provide enzymes that your body may not make or that you do not make enough of. This step alone can have a profound, positive effect on digestion and the reversal of leaky gut syndrome.

The next step is adding omega-3 fatty acids, which can help to reduce inflammation by halting the cascade of arachidonic acid. By reducing inflammation in this manner, intestinal healing will progress more quickly. It is important to note that this step also has a profound effect on ADHD in general. By removing inflammation within the brain and nervous system, the symptoms of ADHD can be significantly reduced.

The final step in healing the gut is the use of probiotics, which help increase the amount of beneficial bacteria and yeast in the intestinal tract. These microbes further help break down your food and also prevent the colonization of unfriendly bacteria that contribute to poor gastrointestinal health. Because both friendly and unfriendly microbes use the same food sources, a high level of friendly bacteria in the gut can prevent unfriendly bacteria from colonizing by essentially starving them of their food source. It is important to note that the primary food source for these microbes is sugar. So if the diet is high in sugar, both the friendly and unfriendly microbes will feast and flourish. Therefore, to have the greatest positive effect on gastrointestinal flora, greatly limit sugar consumption and reduce carbohydrate consumption in general, as carbohydrates are easily broken down into sugars during digestion. Most children with ADHD have been found to have abnormal cortisol rhythms, a condition that is frequently associated with poor carbohydrate metabolism, resulting in an even greater need to limit sugar intake.

While leaky gut syndrome is definitely one of the most profoundly negative outcomes of a diet that includes gluten and dairy products, it is not the only consequence. In addition to promoting a leaky gut, gluten and dairy products are high in certain proteins called lectins, which adversely affect the nervous system.

Lectins are proteins that bind to carbohydrates, usually on cell membranes. The cell membrane is a site of heavy activity, as this is where the cell determines whether or not a molecule can enter. When this activity is compromised, the cell no longer functions properly. Lectins bind to cell membranes and disrupt this activity; depending on the degree of dysfunction that is caused, it could lead to cell death.

This is particularly noteworthy for the cells of the nervous system, as their primary activity is to create a synaptic potential (also called nerve cell firings). All information within the nervous system is transmitted via a carefully orchestrated series of synaptic potentials. A synaptic potential is only allowed to occur if certain channels on the cell membrane are able to properly open and close, allowing electrolytes, such as calcium and potassium, to cross the cell membrane and create an electrochemical charge. When the cell membrane is not working properly, this electrochemical charge does not occur appropriately. This could mean that the nerve cells fire when they shouldn't or don't fire when they should. In either case, the nervous system is compromised, resulting in a variety of possible neurological dysfunctions, including ADHD. Gluten and dairy products are both high in the lectins that have been directly implicated in ADHD.

When looking at the big picture and seeing how gluten and dairy products negatively affect the body and mind in so many disparate ways, it seems like an easy decision to remove these foods from our diets. Fortunately, we live in a time when gluten-free and dairy-free substitutes for almost any food are readily available at your local natural food store. Even if ADHD affects only your child, you may find that when you remove these foods from your diet along with your child's diet, any symptoms that you may be experiencing will be reduced as well.

ADHD and the Thyroid Gland

If your child is showing symptoms that you think may be attention deficit hyperactivity disorder, don't be so fast to apply that label. There are other conditions that can produce similar symptoms. Before jumping to conclusions, rule out a possible thyroid problem.

While ADHD is the most commonly diagnosed behavioral disorder in children, there are no specific laboratory tests to confirm the diagnosis. The diagnosis is determined by the presence of a variety of symptoms that can include, to varying degrees, inattentiveness, difficulty concentrating, distractibility, hyperactivity, and impulsive behavior. Not everyone with an ADHD diagnosis need display all of these behaviors. Children, especially girls with the inattentive form of ADHD, are often not diagnosed until middle school because of their lack of disruptive behavior. Others may be hyperactive and impulsive but not necessarily inattentive. Recent studies have demonstrated a physiologic basis for this difference.

The thyroid gland produces hormones that are essential for normal brain development. In children, often the earliest indications of an overactive thyroid, called hyperthyroidism, may be behavioral as opposed to physical. Nervousness, a key hyperthyroid symptom, may be expressed in children as hyperactivity. Moodiness, forgetfulness, and inattention are also common symptoms of hyperthyroidism and all are common features of ADHD as well. Due to a specific gene mutation, some people show a reduced responsiveness to the thyroid hormones, a condition known as generalized resistance to thyroid hormone, or GRTH. Although not a particularly common disorder, about 70 percent of children with this genetic resistance to thyroid hormone exhibit symptoms of ADHD. Furthermore, children with GRTH are more prone to learning disabilities than children with ADHD.

The typical laboratory picture of hyperthyroidism will show high levels of the thyroid hormones triiodothyronine (T3) and thyroxine (T4) and a low level of thyroid stimulating hormone (TSH), which is produced by the pituitary gland and stimulates the thyroid gland when the body senses that more thyroid hormone is needed. In GRTH, levels of T3 and T4 will be high, as in regular hyperthyroidism, but TSH levels will be normal to high.

Researchers studying this phenomenon have shown that the high levels of T3 and T4 are significantly correlated with symptoms of hyperactivity and impulsivity but do not seem to have any correlation to symptoms of inattention or distractibility. Levels of TSH do not correlate significantly with any of the symptoms of ADHD.

When evaluating the thyroid gland to see if it may be involved as a cause of behavioral symptoms similar to ADHD, be suspicious if the lab results don't fit the clinical picture. There have been cases where an unusual antibody that reacts with the standard TSH test gives a false high reading, suggestive of GRTH, when in fact the TSH is actually low.

Given the frustration, not to mention the expense, of evaluating and treating children with ADHD, it makes sense to screen for thyroid problems first, using simple, noninvasive, readily available tests.

To Medicate or Not to Medicate

There is no drug that can cure ADHD. Prescription drugs may suppress some of the symptoms, but not without many potentially serious side effects, and ADHD drugs are prescribed for long-term use. Even if your child is experiencing side effects from prescribed medication, it's important to never discontinue stimulants or antidepressants without first consulting your health care professional. The withdrawal symptoms can be more severe than the adverse reactions to these medications. Therefore, the process must be closely monitored by a mental health professional.

Ritalin has been associated with sleeplessness, addiction, depression, and other unpleasant consequences. At the beginning of the treatment, the side effects can be quite serious. Besides changing the child's behavior from unruliness to docility, making him more socially acceptable, Ritalin can cause nausea, vomiting, mood swings, loss of appetite, decreased height, and weight loss. Here are some facts about Ritalin and other drugs commonly prescribed to treat ADHD:

- The government estimates that 2.5 million American children and 1.5 million American adults take medication for ADHD.
- The side effects reported on Ritalin's label include stomachaches, headaches, and hallucinations, but reports have suggested it also causes more severe reactions, such as liver problems and even death. The FDA's advisory committee voted eight to seven in favor of putting a black box warning—the FDA's most severe warning for side effects in drugs—on the box of Ritalin, but the FDA has not yet taken any action on the recommendation. This was after data revealed that ADHD drugs may have caused twenty-five deaths and fifty-four serious medical problems among patients between the years 1999 and 2003. Cited medical problems include stroke, hypertension, palpitations, arrhythmia, and heart attacks.

- Between the years 1990 and 2000, more than 569 children were hospitalized. Thirty-eight of these incidences were life-threatening and 186 children died, all from using stimulants. Many of them died from cardiac arrest and strokes.
- All stimulants cause constriction of veins and arteries, causing the heart to work overtime, leading to damage to the heart.
- Victoria Vetter, a pediatric cardiologist at the University of Pennsylvania School of Medicine and the head of the heart group committee, recommends that children should have an EKG to rule out any undiagnosed heart issues before they are put on pharmaceuticals. She said that after screening 1,100 children, she found that 2 percent of them had some type of heart problem.
- Schools receive additional money from the state and federal governments for every child labeled with ADHD and prescribed medication.
- Children twelve years and older who have been prescribed or are currently taking any stimulants or antidepressants are automatically rejected for military service.
- Amphetamines, such as Dexedrine and Adderall, are toxic to the brain and can cause brain cell death. In several studies with lab animals, such as rhesus monkeys, small doses of amphetamines were administered over periods of days or weeks. The animals showed a lasting loss of receptors for the neurotransmitter dopamine.
- Ritalin is highly addictive. It's a Schedule II category drug, along with morphine, cocaine, opium, and barbiturates. Common street names for Ritalin include rids, pineapple, and kiddie cocaine.
- No studies have been conducted on Ritalin for children under six years old.
- Strattera is the newest drug that Eli Lilly and Company is promoting for ADHD. It's been dispensed to more than two million patients since it went on the market in 2002. Eli Lilly and Company was required to include a black box warning on the package.

In some children and teens, Strattera increases the risk of suicidal thoughts. A combined analysis of twelve studies of Strattera showed that in children and teens this risk was 0.4 percent for those taking Strattera compared to none for those taking a sugar pill. A similar analysis in adults treated with Strattera did not reveal an increased risk of suicidal thoughts. Call your doctor right away if your child has thoughts of suicide or sudden changes in mood or behavior, especially at the beginning of treatment or after a change in dose.

Naturopathy and ADHD

Naturopathic doctors (NDs) are trained as primary care physicians who specialize in treating a variety of health conditions using natural therapies. They are considered to be a bridge between conventional and traditional medicine and have extensive experience treating patients suffering from ADHD and other neurological disorders.

After completing four years of postgraduate schooling at one of only six accredited naturopathic medical colleges in North America, naturopathic physicians must earn their board certification prior to becoming licensed to practice medicine. The following are the six principles followed by naturopathic physicians:

1. First, do no harm.
2. Identify and treat causes.
3. Let nature heal.
4. Treat the whole person.
5. Educate patients.
6. Prevent illness.

Depending on the state in which an ND practices, some of these doctors are able to prescribe pharmaceutical drugs. However, naturopathic philosophy dictates that natural, holistic treatments be used initially. These treatments include the use of herbs, nutrients, homeopathic remedies, dietary changes, physical medicine, and hydrotherapy, just to name a few. The treatment chosen depends entirely on the individual's health status along with his or her current health challenges. Many chronic conditions unresponsive to conventional (allopathic) therapies often improve when treated with naturopathy.

The healing approach of an ND involves determining a "cause" for a specific illness and then treating or removing that cause, as opposed to merely masking symptoms with medication. These well-trained doctors use standard testing methods, such as X-rays, blood tests, physical exams, ultrasound, and other diagnostic techniques to arrive at the source of a patient's illness. Once the root cause has been removed, optimal wellness may be achieved. This approach can be used to treat illnesses ranging from allergies and asthma to heart disease and cancers.

A naturopathic physician uses this approach in treating ADHD. The approach begins with ordering diagnostic tests, which might include obtaining stool samples to determine the presence of yeast overgrowth, standard blood tests to determine the overall health and nutritional status of the patient, and organic amino acid tests. Once a cause has been established, an individualized treatment plan is developed to help remove the cause. Typically this is done through the use of herbal treatments, nutritional supplementation, dietary modifications, or homeopathic remedies. In the case of ADHD, the culprit is often determined to be a food sensitivity or sensitivity to a particular preservative or food dye. By removing the offending item, many children diagnosed with ADHD show marked improvement in their behavior.

When treating children with autism, NDs often incorporate therapies that support the child's immune system. This might include improving digestion by eliminating yeast overgrowth, using homeopathic remedies that help antidote adverse reactions to vaccines, and prescribing supplements to improve nutritional status.

A therapy that is often used when treating ADHD is called craniosacral therapy. This hands-on treatment was developed by an osteopathic physician.

During a craniosacral therapy session, the patient lies fully clothed on his or her back while the practitioner uses a series of gentle maneuvers to help restore balance to the lymphatic system. After a few moments, the patient enters a state of relaxation caused by a natural parasympathetic response of the body to this hands-on technique. The parasympathetic nervous system is a division of the autonomic nervous system, and it's responsible for promoting a restful state in addition to promoting digestion. Its counterpart is the sympathetic nervous system, which is responsible for causing a "fight or flight" response. So it's easy to see how invoking a restful state would be beneficial when treating ADHD. But craniosacral therapy goes well beyond merely invoking a parasympathetic state. It also assists in removing blockages throughout the body. Many practitioners believe that the combined effects of craniosacral therapy serve as a useful adjunct to other naturopathic treatments for ADHD.

Homeopathy and ADHD

Homeopathy is essentially an energetic treatment method based on the belief that matter and energy are the same, existing in different forms and subject to change. Homeopathic remedies help to exert a positive constitutional change, and the results are possibly due to unobserved quantum effects. The homeopathic system is based on the principle that diseases can be cured with minute doses of medicines, which in a healthy person in large doses would produce symptoms like those of the disease. Homeopathy has been practiced for over two hundred years and is not a new treatment method or medical craze.

Homeopathic medicines are dilutions prepared from many natural substances, mainly herbs. But there are also remedies prepared from animal and bacterial tissues. The remedies are made by successive dilutions, meaning they are diluted with water, and then a drop from the dilution is again mixed with a certain amount of water, and so on. At each step of dilution, the substance is shaken (succussed) a number of times to reach the desired potency. The more the remedy is diluted, the more powerful it becomes, though it is not yet understood exactly why.

The reason homeopathy is so effective is that it treats the whole person and not the disease. Homeopaths do not diagnose. Rather, they prescribe remedies based on a symptom overview provided by the patient, which covers all aches and pains from head to toe. The overview also includes the mind and emotions and the time of day when conditions are worse. Subjective symptoms are very important. These are often private, secret feelings, but when they are expressed, they become vital clues for determining a remedy.

Homeopathy can be a powerful tool to treat children (as well as adults) suffering from ADHD. As a first aid, homeopathy can treat sleeplessness, anxiety, nervousness, and hyperactivity. An overly impulsive child can be helped with a remedy that makes him stop to think first and act later. For example, there is coffea cruda, which is coffee. When given in a microdose, coffee is used for sleeplessness. Chamomile is used for the hyperactive child. Arsenicum album and argentum nitricum are used for anxiety and fears. It is advisable not to change remedies too often. Let one bring about the desired result first. Sometimes one remedy acts for a long time.

Since ADHD displays a myriad of symptoms and every person has his or her own unique biochemical makeup, it is important to seek the help of an experienced homeopathic practitioner. Parents should inform themselves about homeopathic medicines before they use any, and the remedies should only be used as first aid. A homeopath should be consulted for constitutional treatments.

The correct remedy is found by checking a multitude of symptoms against a multitude of remedies in what is called the homeopathic repertory and homeopathic materia medica. It takes a lot of skill and expertise on the part of the practitioner to find the correct medicine. But when it is found, it works like a miracle. It happens sometimes that the practitioner has to try several remedies or several different potencies for the patient to achieve the desired state of health, but when the correct remedy is found, the result can be instantaneous.

Homeopathy is gentle and harmless. It does not interfere with any other mode of treatment. You can treat yourself and your children while saving a lot of money. Remedy kits with first aid medicines are available at low cost. These are easy-to-take, small, sweet pellets or tablets. It's best to take them on their own, not with food or drink, preferably at bedtime. Remedies last for a long time and don't lose their effectiveness. They should be stored away from extreme temperatures and strong-smelling chemicals and substances, such as perfume.

Without touching the tablets or pellets, shake four to six of them into the cap that covers the bottle. Put them under the tongue and let them dissolve. Don't eat or drink anything twenty minutes before or after taking them. Make sure your mouth is free of flavors, including mint, coffee, or anything with a strong taste. Although the medicine is best taken at bedtime, any time is acceptable if the above precautions are observed. Always consult with your child's medical doctor before attempting a new treatment.

Tests and Testing Laboratories

Your pediatrician or other doctors may not be familiar with the following tests. The laboratory personnel can consult with your doctor or can provide names of doctors closest to your area who have knowledge of these tests and can provide proper guidance in treating your child. Most of the tests listed are covered by insurance.

Types of Tests
Food and inhalant allergy testing. Children with ADHD often have food allergies, and symptoms worsen after the children eat certain foods. Candi-

diasis (yeast overgrowth) contributes to food allergies. IgG (immunoglobulin) testing shows delayed food sensitivities.

Amino acid deficiencies. Amino acids are the basic building blocks of protein. They form neurotransmitters in the brain that regulate mood and behavior.

Candidiasis. Candidiasis is an overgrowth of yeast and may lead to leaky gut syndrome. Many ADHD and autistic children have tested positive for abnormally high levels of yeast. A gastrointestinal health panel (GI panel) and comprehensive digestive stool analysis (CDSA) are good tests for specific measures of intestinal health that can give rise to yeast, pathogenic bacteria, and parasite overgrowths.

Digestive function. People with ADHD often exhibit chronic digestive problems. A gastrointestinal health panel (GI panel) and comprehensive digestive stool analysis (CDSA) provide the best information to lead to treatment for digestive disorders. Poor digestion can result from an overuse of antibiotics.

Essential fatty acids. Deficiencies in essential fatty acids are very common among children with ADHD.

Heavy metal analysis. People withADHD typically do very well once toxic metals are removed from the body. Urine tests are the most reliable and easiest method to check for heavy metals. Hair testing was popular at one time, but because hair is usually contaminated by cosmetics (such as shampoos) and the environment, it's not an accurate or reliable measurement.

Pesticides and flame-retardant chemicals. All individuals who have symptoms of ADHD should be checked for toxic chemical exposure. This is one of the most overlooked and potentially most important areas of concern because it has a direct and major effect on brain and body chemistry and is relatively easy to correct once the details are known.

Seizures. It is estimated that up to 38 percent of children diagnosed with ADHD have underlying seizures. Testing for amino acids, essential fatty acids, food allergies, environmental toxins, and heavy metals are important for assessing the causes and potential treatment of seizures.

Zinc testing and nutritional testing. Zinc and nutritional deficiencies are common in people with ADHD.

Testing Resources
Diagnos-Techs, Inc.
diagnostechs.com
Tests and services: gastrointestinal health panel.

Doctor's Data, Inc.
doctorsdata.com
Tests and services: urine toxic and essential elements; fecal metals; comprehensive drinking water analysis; yeast culture and sensitivities.

Environmental Health Center—Dallas
ehcd.com
Tests and services: complete blood lab; comprehensive allergy and chemical testing; antigen lab; detoxification sauna; exercise facility; nutritional counseling and education; sauna and massage; environmentally safe facility; purified air and water; toxicological profiles

Genova Diagnostics
gdx.net
Tests and services: genetic testing for problems with detoxification path-

ways; consultations regarding the decision to vaccinate; polypeptide; organic acids; digestive function; intestinal permeability

The Great Plains Laboratory, Inc.

greatplainslaboratory.com

Tests and services: organic acid test for yeast and bacteria overgrowth; vitamin and mineral deficiencies; opiate peptides for gluten and casein sensitivity; toxic exposures to heavy metals; deficiencies in the immune system; abnormal amino acid; comprehensive stool testing

Metametrix Clinical Laboratory

metametrix.com

Tests and services: fatty acids; amino acid profiles; IgE and IgG food antibodies; inhalant antibodies; organic acids test

Pain and Stress Center

painstresscenter.com

Tests and services: nutritional counseling; amino acid testing; food allergy testing; orthomolecular programs; group lectures; educational programs; product research and development; amino acid supplements (call for catalog)

US Biotek Laboratories

usbiotek.com

Tests and services: serum IgG and IgE antibody panels for foods, indoor/outdoor inhalants, spices and herbs; serum or finger stick IgG antibody panels for foods, indoor/outdoor inhalants, spices and herbs; Candida antibodies; serum or finger stick IgG, A, M, and Candida antigen; comprehensive urinary metabolic profile (GC/MS); environmental pollutants panel (GC/MS); high-sensitivity CRP (hs-CRP)

Resources

Clinic

The HANDLE Institute

handle.org

The HANDLE Institute provides an effective, drug-free alternative for identifying and treating most neurodevelopmental disorders, including autism, ADD, ADHD, dyslexia, and Tourette's syndrome.

Household Lead Testing Kits

leadcheck.com

Mercury-Free Dentist Referral Service

International Academy of Oral Medicine and Toxicology

iaomt.org

Naturopathic Physician Locator

The American Association of Naturopathic Physicians

naturopathic.org

Magazines and Newsletters

Alternative Medicine: alternativemedicine.com

Mothering Magazine: mothering.com

Supplements

Child Life Essentials

childlife.net

Nutritional supplements for children and infants.

Montiff

montiff.com

Amino acid and nutritional supplements.

Metabolic Maintenance Products

metabolicmaintenance.com

Customized amino acid formula based on your amino acid profile from any reputable testing laboratory.

Detoxification Products

The American Botanical Pharmacy

herbdoc.com

Dr. Schultz Superfood and intestinal, liver, and gallbladder detoxification herbal formulas.

Bioray, Inc.

bioray.com

Organic supplements for detoxifying from heavy metals and chemicals.

CompliMed

complimed.com

Homeopathic medicines for detoxifying from chemicals, pesticides, and allergens.

Renew Life

renewlife.com

Cleansing products for candidiasis and heavy metals.

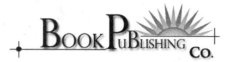

Book Publishing Co.

books that educate, inspire, and empower

Weight Loss and Good Health with **APPLE CIDER VINEGAR** – *Cynthia Holzapfel*

Healthy and Beautiful with **COCONUT OIL** – *Cynthia Holzapfel and Laura Holzapfel*

The Weekend **DETOX** – *Jerry Lee Hutchens*

Improve Digestion with **FOOD COMBINING** – *Steve Meyerowitz*

Understanding **GOUT** – *Warren Jefferson*

PALEO Smoothies – *Alan Roettinger*

Refreshing Fruit and Vegetable **SMOOTHIES** – *Robert Oser*

All titles in the **Live Healthy Now** series are only **$5.95!**

Interested in other health topics or healthy cookbooks?
See our complete line of titles at bookpubco.com or order
directly from:

Book Publishing Company
P.O. Box 99
Summertown, TN 38483
1-888-260-8458